COMPREHEN
THE BAT

A Visionary Method: Exploring
The Advantages Of The Bates
Method

FOSTER GOODNEWS

Copyright © 2023 Foster Goodnews

All rights reserved

Contents

CHAPTER ONE 5

The Bates Approach: A Primer......5

The Bates Approach: Basic Concepts 9

CHAPTER TWO 13

Physiology Of The Eyes...............13

The Roots Of Your Eye Trouble ...16

Gains From The Bates Approach .20

CHAPTER THREE 25

Palming as a Bates Technique.....25

Swinging As A Bates Method Technique 28

Techniques For The Bates Method: Sunbathing 32

CHAPTER FOUR 36

Techniques Used In The Bates Method: Blinking 36

Techniques For The Bates Method Of Exercise 39

Visualization Methods In The Bates Approach 43

CHAPTER FIVE 47

Bates Method Relaxation Exercises 47

Methods For Including The Bates Approach In Your Daily Life 51

Conclusion 55

THE END 58

CHAPTER ONE
The Bates Approach: A Primer

Many vision issues, the theory goes, can be alleviated or even reversed with the use of simple exercises and relaxation techniques to reduce the habitual strain and tension in the eye muscles.

The premise of the Bates Method is that the eyes perform at their peak when they are unrestrained and unrestricted in their range of motion.

The method's exercises and practices are meant to assist people relieve tension in their eye muscles, lessen the effects of eye strain, and sharpen their vision as a whole.

Palming (covering the eyes with the palms of the hands), eye shifting, and sunbathing (exposing the eyes to sunlight) are only a few of the activities included in the Bates Method.

The technique also stresses the significance of practicing healthy eye habits, such as pausing frequently while reading or using a computer to prevent eye strain.

The Bates Method is still debated by conventional eye doctors despite anecdotal proof of its effectiveness. However, other studies have not demonstrated any substantial improvement in vision using this strategy.

Before trying the Bates Method or any other vision rehabilitation program, it is vital to speak with a qualified healthcare expert, as is the case with any alternative therapy.

The Bates Approach: Basic Concepts

The Bates Method's exercises and techniques are grounded in a number of principles. Principles such as these are:

• The Bates Method, which aims to improve eyesight, places an emphasis on relaxing the eyes. Blurred vision can be caused by tension and worry in the eyes, thus learning to relax the eyes and the mind is an important part of the process.

• The Bates Method, which emphasizes eye exercises and

practices designed to minimize strain on the eyes, supports the belief that healthy vision is a natural state that can be restored.

- The approach places a premium on central fixation, or the capacity to maintain attention on a single point in space. Central fixation training has been shown to enhance visual acuity and alleviate eye fatigue.

- The Bates Method contains exercises designed to encourage the natural movement and shifting of focus of the eyes, as is their design. To increase their range of motion and flexibility, the eyes can benefit from eye workouts like palming, eye shifting, and sunbathing.

• The Bates Method recommends healthy practices for your eyes, such as taking regular pauses from reading or computer use, getting plenty of rest, and never letting your eyes stay open for too long.

The overall goal of the Bates Method is to improve eyesight and reduce eye strain by encouraging relaxation, natural movement, and good habits.

CHAPTER TWO
Physiology Of The Eyes

The eyes are a pair of intricate organs that coordinate their functions to allow humans to see. An outline of the eyes' operation is as follows:

• The cornea is the transparent outer layer of the eye that allows light to enter the eye. Light is focused by the cornea onto the lens.

• The lens, which sits behind the iris (the eye's colored component), changes shape so that light can be focused onto the retina.

• Back at the back of the eye is a layer of specialized cells called the retina, which processes the light and sends electrical signals via the optic nerve to the brain.

• The visual world is converted from a series of electrical signals into a mental image by the brain.

Muscles in the eye sockets also allow us to change our eye's shape and focus on objects at varying distances, as well as follow moving targets.

The eyes also include rods and cones, which are responsible for low-light vision and color perception, respectively. Our central vision and visual acuity come from a little spot in the center of the retina called the macula.

The eyes, as a system, are very intricate and crucial to our capacity to see and understand the environment.

The Roots Of Your Eye Trouble

Vision impairments can have multiple causes. Some typical explanations include:

• Myopia, hyperopia, and astigmatism are all examples of refractive errors, which occur when the eye's shape improperly bends light and blurs vision.

• Vision loss can occur as a result of age-related changes in the eyes. Many adults over the age of 40 suffer from presbyopia, an eye disorder brought on by the lens's decreasing adaptability.

- Cataracts, glaucoma, and macular degeneration are all examples of eye illnesses that, if left untreated, can lead to impaired vision or possibly blindness.

- Injuries to the eye can cause a wide spectrum of vision issues, from mild irritation to permanent blindness.

- Color blindness and some forms of refractive defects, for example, can run in families.

- Eyestrain and other visual difficulties can be caused by environmental factors such as long periods of exposure to bright sunshine or computer screens.

• Systemic disorders: Diabetes and high blood pressure are two examples of systemic diseases that can have an impact on the eyes and lead to visual impairment.

Having your eyes checked on a routine basis can help catch visual issues early so they can be treated. Glasses, contact lenses, or even surgery may be able to help or completely correct a person's eyesight.

Gains From The Bates Approach

The Bates Method is an approach to better eyesight that does not include corrective lenses of any kind, prescription or otherwise. Among the possible advantages of the Bates Method are:

• By relieving tension in the eye muscles, the Bates Method is said to improve clarity of vision. Those who suffer from nearsightedness (myopia), farsightedness (astigmatism), or presbyopia (age-related farsightedness) may benefit greatly from this.

• The Bates Method was developed to relieve the strain on one's eyes caused by staring at a computer screen for long periods of time or performing other visually demanding tasks. Learning to relax the eyes can help reduce eye strain and headaches.

• The Bates Method includes eye exercises specifically developed to improve cross-eye coordination. People with vision problems like double vision or poor depth perception may find this useful.

• The Bates Method stresses the value of gaining a deeper

understanding of one's own visual habits and patterns. Learning to be more self-aware about our eye use can help us break bad habits that put unnecessary pressure on our eyes.

• While the Bates Method does not guarantee that it will fully eliminate the need for corrective lenses, it may help some people lessen their dependency on glasses or contact lenses.

However, some medical professionals may question the efficacy of the Bates Method and it should be noted that this is not a consensus. Before beginning any new health or wellness routine, it is wise to discuss the plan with a trusted medical professional.

CHAPTER THREE
Palming as a Bates Technique

The Bates Method employs a relaxing method called palming,

which is placing one's palms over one's eyes to create a warm, dark atmosphere in which to rest one's eyes. The procedure for palming is as follows:

• Relax in a chair and prop up your elbows on a nearby surface.

• Warm up your hands by rubbing them together vigorously for a few seconds.

• Put your hands together palms up, and close your eyes, being careful not to press on your eyeballs while you do so.

• Put your shoulders back and your neck straight, and take calm, deep breaths.

• Try focusing on the blackness, or on a calming image or recollection.

• You should rest with your palms over your eyes for 5-10 minutes, or as long as you feel relaxed.

• Slowly take your hands off your face and open your eyes when you are ready.

People who spend extended periods of time staring at a computer screen or indulging in other visually demanding activities may find palming to be useful in relieving eye strain and promoting relaxation. If you want to see improvements, you should do palming at least twice a day.

Swinging As A Bates Method Technique

The Bates Method includes a swinging exercise for better eye coordination and less strain on the eyes. The procedure for swinging is as follows:

• Maintain a comfortable stance with your feet hip-width apart and your arms at your sides.

- Focus your attention on something out of the room, like a tree or a building.

- Swing your whole body from side to side instead of just your head to let your eyes track the thing as it moves across your field of vision.

- Keep your eyes moving and your breathing normal while you swing.

- Keep swinging for several minutes, working up to faster speeds and wider swings.

- Stop swinging and close your eyes for a moment as you breathe deeply to calm down.

The goal of swinging is to strengthen the muscles of the visual system and increase eye-hand coordination. Swinging for a few minutes multiple times day, or as often as needed, can help reduce eye strain. However, before trying swinging or any other Bates Method approach, it is crucial to consult with a knowledgeable healthcare expert, as is the case with any new exercise or wellness practice.

Techniques For The Bates Method: Sunbathing

Bates Method practitioners often resort to sunbathing as a means of relaxation. The procedure for tanning is as follows:

• Locate a comfortable outdoor seating area in the sun.

• Put your eyes out of your mind and loosen up your face.

• Face the sun, taking care not to stare directly at it or subject your eyes to prolonged exposure to bright light.

• Close your eyes and imagine the sun's rays penetrating them and bathing your eyes with their restorative radiance.

• Take a few slow, deep breaths and tune in to how the sun's rays feel against your skin.

• Keep tanning for a little longer; as you become used to it, you can up the time spent in the sun.

• Turn your face away from the sun and slowly open your eyes when you are ready. This will give your eyes time to acclimate to the brightness.

The sun's rays are thought to ease tension in the eyes and help them rest easier. To get the most out of tanning, it is advisable to do it daily, preferably twice. However, before trying sunbathing or any other Bates Method approach, it is crucial to speak with a trained healthcare expert, as is the case with any new workout or wellness practice.

CHAPTER FOUR
Techniques Used In The Bates Method: Blinking

The Bates Method to help people with poor eyesight. Blinking is an important part of this strategy. This is how it functions:

• The Bates Method emphasizes the importance of blinking as a means to relieve eye strain and calm the nervous system. Our eyes get a much-needed bath in a solution of lubricating tears every time we blink. Maintaining healthy eyes requires natural tears, and blinking helps increase their production.

• In order to improve your eyesight by blinking, you should make it a habit to blink regularly throughout the day, and especially when engaging in visually demanding tasks like reading, using a computer, or driving. Maintain a rate of one blink every five seconds, and make it a point to completely close your eyelids when you do so.

• To further relax your eyes, you can also practice "palming" in addition to the frequent blinking you already do during the day. Palming involves covering closed eyelids with palms while keeping fingers out of the way. Close your eyes and let your thoughts wander while you palm for a while.

Blinking is an easy way to alleviate eye strain and boost visual acuity. To maintain eye health and enhance vision naturally, try to blink more often and incorporate regular palming into your routine.

Techniques For The Bates Method Of Exercise

Shifting is another tool used in the Bates Method to enhance vision; it entails making movements that loosen up the muscles in your eyes and make them more adaptable. Here's the procedure:

• Pick something out of the way, like a tree or a structure, and concentrate on it with your eyes.

• Do not move your head, but try focusing on anything closer by, like a leaf on a tree.

• Then, return your attention to the original faraway thing.

• Alternate between the far and near object multiple times, repeating the shifting exercise each time.

The flexing and relaxing of the eye muscles is facilitated by this shifting exercise. Training your eyes to focus at various distances and on various objects can also assist enhance your eyesight as a whole.

Other objects at varying distances, such as a book at arm's length and a picture on the wall, can be used for this practice as well. The trick is to make a concerted effort to switch gears effortlessly through regular practice.

Shifting is an easy method that helps with eyesight and reduces strain on the eyes. You can assist maintain good eye health and perhaps enhance your eyesight by making this a regular part of your regimen.

Visualization Methods In The Bates Approach

The Bates Method incorporates visual imagery as another strategy for correcting vision issues. By conjuring up images in your head, you may sharpen your focus and see things more clearly. Here's the procedure:

• Pick an Item: Pick an item that you can easily picture in your mind. A writing on a page, an image on a wall, or a far-off landscape are all examples.

• Put your focus on the image in your mind's eye and close your eyes. See if you can get as much clarity and specificity out of it as you can.

• Imagine the object in your mind so that it is clearer, brighter, and more vivid than it is in reality. Picture the colors to be more vibrant, the lines to be sharper, and the details to be clearer.

• Do this visualisation practice regularly, ideally multiple times per day.

By fortifying the neural pathways linking the two, visualization enhances one's capacity to process visual data. Seeing things more clearly in your mind's eye can help you see them more clearly in the real world.

Visualization can also be used to sharpen one's depth perception, color vision, or peripheral vision. You can improve these features of your vision over time by focusing on envisioning them as sharper and more defined.

Visualizing positive outcomes for one's eyesight and relieving tension on one's eyes is a straightforward yet efficient method. You can assist maintain good eye health and perhaps enhance your eyesight by making this a regular part of your regimen.

CHAPTER FIVE
Bates Method Relaxation Exercises

The Bates Method for Eye Improvement emphasizes relaxation as a means to better vision. The eyes and their surrounding muscles can benefit from less strain and increased blood flow if you learn to relax them. The Bates Method employs the following methods of stress reduction:

• Palming is when you close your eyes and cover them with your palms without letting your fingers touch your eyes. The muscles in your eye area will unwind and you will not have to struggle to see well. The best conditions for palming are complete silence and low lighting.

• Relaxation techniques like deep breathing exercises can help alleviate stress and tension anywhere in the body, including the eyes. Take long, leisurely breaths in through your nose and out through your mouth as a simple breathing exercise. Pay attention to your breathing, and with each exhale, consciously relax a muscle.

• Reducing tension in your eyes might also help you relax your body. One technique is to lie down in a relaxed position and, beginning with the toes, slowly move the focus up the body. Hold a tense position for a few seconds, then relax.

• Relaxing your mind and relieving strain on your eyes are both possible through the practice of visualization. Think of a tranquil place, like a beach or a forest, and picture yourself unwinding with every passing second.

Regular practice of these stress-reduction methods has been shown to have beneficial effects on eye health, including a reduction in the effects of eye strain. Reduce stress and boost your health by making relaxing a regular part of your routine.

Methods For Including The Bates Approach In Your Daily Life

Using the Bates Method regularly? Here are some suggestions.

- Beginning with just one or two Bates Method practices, like palming or visualization, in your everyday routine is a great place to start. As you gain experience with these methods, you can incorporate more ones.

- Practice the Bates Method practices regularly and you will see results. Make sure to practice often, even if it is just for a few minutes a day.

- Do things like palming exercises on your lunch break or mental imagery drills before bed as part of your regular routine to reinforce the benefits of the Bates Method. You have a better chance of maintaining these practices if you see them as routine.

• Maintain a calm demeanor and rest your eyes while performing Bates Method exercises. Take a break if you need to, and come back to it later if you are still having trouble.

• To correct your vision with the Bates Method, you must be patient. Trust that with regular practice, your eyesight will progressively improve over time, even if you do not perceive any changes right away.

• If you are new to the Bates Method and want to be sure you are doing it right, it is a good idea to find a certified practitioner or teacher to help you get started.

The Bates Method can be used to improve eye health and vision in a more natural way. Your eyesight can gradually improve if you are consistent and patient.

Conclusion

The Bates Method is a non-invasive alternative to corrective lenses, surgery, and/or eyewear designed to improve eyesight naturally.

The Bates Method is an attempt to alleviate eye strain by increasing blood flow to the eyes and decreasing the amount of time spent looking at a single point of focus.

Although there is no scientific evidence that the Bates Method improves eyesight, many people have claimed to see benefits with regular use.

If you are interested in giving the Bates Method a try, you should only do so under the supervision of a trained professional.

The Bates Method is a holistic and natural way to improve your eyesight that can be used in conjunction with conventional techniques. The Bates Method can be used to maintain healthy eyes and gradually enhance one's eyesight through simple, everyday practices.

THE END

Printed in Great Britain
by Amazon